C000091149

HIGH FIBER VEGETARIAN COOKBOOK

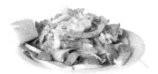

Delicious Low Fat and Plant Based Recipes to Manage Diabetes, High Cholesterol, High Blood Pressure, and IBS and Enhance Your Well-being

Dr. Mary D. Torres

DISCLAIMER

The High Fiber Vegetarian Cookbook is a collection of recipes and dietary guidelines intended to support individuals managing Diabetes, High blood pressure and High Cholesterol. While every effort has been made to ensure the accuracy and reliability of the information presented, it is essential to note that this cookbook is not a substitute for professional medical advice, diagnosis, or treatment.

Readers are strongly advised to consult with a qualified healthcare professional or registered dietitian before making significant changes to their diet, especially if they are managing specific medical conditions, such as diabetes. The recipes and nutritional information provided in this cookbook are general recommendations and may not be suitable for everyone.

Individuals with food allergies, sensitivities, or dietary restrictions should exercise caution and carefully review the ingredient lists, considering their unique health circumstances. The authors, publishers, and contributors of this cookbook cannot be held responsible for any adverse effects, reactions, or consequences resulting from the use of the recipes or information contained herein.

The goal of this cookbook is to provide inspiration and guidance for crafting high fiber meals, but individual health requirements may vary.

By using this cookbook, readers acknowledge and agree to the terms of this disclaimer.

Table of Contents

INTRODUCTION

In a world where you can live healthy with proper dietary choices, imagine your body as a finely tuned machine, its gears slowing down due to the repercussions of a low-fiber diet. Picture the sluggishness, the imbalance, and the toll it takes on your overall well-being. This is a call for a High Fiber Vegetarian Diet Cookbook. In this cookbook we embark on a transformative journey toward vitality and health.

This cookbook is beyond compilation of recipes, it's a natural guide to rekindling the symbiotic relationship between flavor and nourishment. In the pages of this culinary inspiration, we weave a narrative of plant-based living, underscoring the profound impact a high fiber vegetarian diet can have on the body. Each dish is crafted with purpose, offering not just delicious alternatives but a pathway to managing and overcoming health challenges.

If you are grappling with diabetes, high cholesterol, and high blood pressure, this cookbook serves as a beacon of culinary hope. The recipes are meticulously designed to not only tantalize taste buds but also to address specific health needs. We delve into the scientific underpinnings of plant-based nutrition, explaining how fiber-rich ingredients can play a pivotal role in managing these conditions.

From breakfasts that set the tone for a vibrant day to dinners that redefine the art of nutritious indulgence, I invite you to rediscover the joy of eating well. Whether you're a seasoned plant-based enthusiast or taking your first steps toward a healthier lifestyle, this cookbook is your compass.

The journey within these pages extends beyond the kitchen, offering insights into mindful eating, nutritional wisdom, and the joy of creating meals that heal. This cookbook is a celebration of the marriage between flavor and well-being, an ode to the transformative power of a high fiber vegetarian diet. Embrace this culinary adventure, where each recipe is a step towards reclaiming the vitality that is rightfully yours.

CHAPTER 1: BASICS OF HIGH FIBER DIET

Definition of High Fiber Foods?

High fiber foods are dietary sources that are rich in fiber, they are type of carbohydrate that the body cannot digest. Instead of being broken down into nutrients and absorbed, fiber passes through the digestive system relatively intact, providing a range of health benefits. There are two main types of dietary fiber: soluble and insoluble.

Soluble Fiber:

Description: Soluble fiber dissolves in water to form a gel-like substance. It can help lower blood cholesterol levels and regulate blood sugar levels.

Sources: Oats, barley, legumes (beans and lentils), fruits (especially apples, citrus fruits, and berries), vegetables (such as carrots and Brussels sprouts), and flaxseeds.

Insoluble Fiber:

Description: Insoluble fiber does not dissolve in water and adds bulk to the stool, promoting regular bowel movements and preventing constipation.

Sources: Whole grains (brown rice, whole wheat, quinoa), nuts and seeds, vegetables (especially broccoli, celery, and dark leafy greens), and the skins of fruits.

Key Points:

Digestive Health: Both types of fiber contribute to digestive health by promoting regular bowel movements, preventing constipation, and supporting a healthy gut microbiome.

Weight Management: High fiber foods are often low in calories which provide a feeling of fullness, thus, making them beneficial for weight management by reducing overall calorie intake.

Blood Sugar Control: Soluble fiber can help regulate blood sugar levels by slowing the absorption of sugar and improving insulin sensitivity.

Heart Health: Soluble fiber has been linked to lower cholesterol levels, and help reduce the risk of heart disease and stroke.

Disease Prevention: A diet rich in high fiber foods has been associated with a lower risk of various chronic diseases, including certain types of cancer (such as colorectal cancer) and type 2 diabetes.

Blood Pressure: Some studies suggest that a high fiber diet may contribute to lower blood pressure levels.

Benefits of a Plant-Based Diet for Health

A plant-based diet which is characterized by the emphasis on whole, plant-derived foods and the exclusion or limited consumption of animal products, offers a myriad of health benefits. There are several key advantages associated with adopting a plant-based lifestyle but let's take a discussion at few of them:

Heart Health:

Plant-based diets are often rich in fiber, antioxidants, and phytochemicals, this contribute to lower levels of cholesterol and blood pressure. This can reduce the risk of cardiovascular diseases.

Weight Management:

Plant-based diets are typically lower in calories and saturated fats, this makes them more effective for weight management. The abundance of fiber also promotes a feeling of fullness, reducing overeating.

Type 2 Diabetes Prevention and Management:

Plant-based diets have been linked to improved insulin sensitivity and lower risk of type 2 diabetes. The high fiber content helps regulate blood sugar levels.

Cancer Risk Reduction:

A plant-based diet, especially one rich in fruits, vegetables, and whole grains, has been associated with a lower risk of certain cancers, including colorectal, breast, and prostate cancers.

Digestive Health:

The fiber content in plant-based foods supports a healthy digestive system, this help in preventing constipation and promoting regular bowel movements. It also contributes to a diverse and beneficial gut microbiome.

Anti-Inflammatory Effects:

Many plant-based foods have anti-inflammatory properties due to their rich content of antioxidants and other bioactive compounds. Chronic inflammation is linked to various diseases, and a plant-based diet may help mitigate this.

Improved Blood Sugar Control:

Plant-based diets, particularly those emphasizing whole foods, have been shown to enhance glycemic control, which makes them beneficial for individuals with diabetes or at risk of developing the condition.

Lower Blood Pressure:

The potassium-rich nature of many plant foods, along with the absence of high-sodium processed foods contributes to lower blood pressure levels.

Improved Gut Health:

Plant-based diets, abundant in fiber and prebiotics, support a healthy gut microbiome. A diverse and balanced microbiome is associated with better overall health and immune function.

Longevity:

Studies have suggested that adherence to a plant-based diet is linked to increased life expectancy, likely due to the combination of various health benefits associated with this eating pattern.

Importance of Managing Diabetes, High Cholesterol, High Blood Pressure, and IBS through Diet

Managing diabetes, high cholesterol, high blood pressure, and irritable bowel syndrome (IBS) through diet is of paramount importance, as these chronic conditions significantly impact health and well-being. Below is breakdown of the importance of dietary management for each condition:

Diabetes:

Blood Sugar Control: A well-managed diet is important for individuals with diabetes to regulate blood sugar levels. By monitoring carbohydrate intake, choosing complex carbs with high fiber content, and incorporating lean proteins contribute to better glycemic control.

High Cholesterol:

Heart Health: Dietary choices play a key role in managing cholesterol levels. A heart-healthy diet low in saturated and trans fats, and rich in soluble fiber can help lower LDL (bad) cholesterol and reduce the risk of cardiovascular diseases.

High Blood Pressure:

Sodium Reduction: Dietary strategies are fundamental in controlling high blood pressure. Limiting sodium intake, increasing potassium-rich foods, and adopting a diet rich in fruits, vegetables, and whole grains contribute to blood pressure management.

Irritable Bowel Syndrome (IBS):

Symptom Management: Diet plays a critical role in alleviating symptoms of IBS. First is to Identify and avoid trigger foods, incorporate soluble fiber to regulate bowel movements, and maintaining a balanced diet can help manage discomfort associated with IBS.

Cross-Cutting Importance:

Weight Management:

Obesity Connection: Effective dietary management contributes to weight control, which is crucial for preventing and managing diabetes, high cholesterol, and high blood pressure. Maintaining a healthy weight also reduces the risk of complications associated with these conditions.

Inflammation Reduction:

Anti-Inflammatory Diet: Chronic conditions often involve inflammation. Adopting an anti-inflammatory diet, rich in fruits, vegetables, and omega-3 fatty acids, may help mitigate inflammation associated with diabetes, high cholesterol, and other chronic diseases.

Overall Well-being:

Nutrient-Rich Foods: A balanced, nutrient-dense diet supports overall well-being. Essential nutrients from a variety of foods contribute to energy, immune function, and the body's ability to heal and recover.

Medication Support:

Enhancing Medication Efficacy: Dietary choices can complement the effects of medications. For example, a heart-healthy diet can enhance the effectiveness of cholesterol-lowering medications, and blood pressure management through diet may support antihypertensive medications.

CHAPTER 2: BREAKFAST DELIGHTS

1. Avocado and Chickpea Toast

Benefits: Packed with healthy fats and fiber, this breakfast promotes heart health, regulates blood sugar, and supports digestive health.

Ingredients:

1 ripe avocado

1/2 cup cooked chickpeas

Whole grain toast

Cherry tomatoes, sliced

Salt and pepper to taste

Preparation:

Mash the avocado and spread it on whole grain toast.

Top with cooked chickpeas and sliced cherry tomatoes.

Sprinkle with salt and pepper to taste.

2. Berry and Chia Seed Parfait

Benefits: Rich in antioxidants and omega-3 fatty acids, this parfait is an excellent choice for managing cholesterol and supporting overall cardiovascular health.

Ingredients:

1 cup mixed berries (strawberries, blueberries, raspberries)

2 tablespoons chia seeds

1 cup plant-based yogurt

1 tablespoon maple syrup (optional)

Granola for topping

Preparation:

In a bowl, mix chia seeds with plant-based yogurt and let it sit for 10 minutes.

Layer the chia-yogurt mixture with mixed berries.

Drizzle with maple syrup if desired and top with granola.

3. Spinach and Mushroom Scramble

Benefits: A low-fat, protein-packed breakfast that supports blood pressure regulation and provides essential nutrients.

Ingredients:

1 cup spinach, chopped

1/2 cup mushrooms, sliced

1/2 block firm tofu, crumbled

1 teaspoon turmeric

Salt and pepper to taste

Whole grain tortilla

Preparation:

Sauté spinach and mushrooms until wilted.

Add crumbled tofu, turmeric, salt, and pepper. Cook until heated through.

Serve in a whole grain tortilla.

4. Oatmeal with Walnuts and Berries

Benefits: Oats contribute to lower cholesterol, and walnuts provide omega-3 fatty acids for heart health.

Ingredients:

1/2 cup old-fashioned oats

1 cup plant-based milk

1 tablespoon chopped walnuts

Mixed berries for topping

1 tablespoon maple syrup (optional)

Preparation:

Cook oats with plant-based milk according to package instructions.

Top with chopped walnuts, mixed berries, and a drizzle of maple syrup if desired.

5. Quinoa Breakfast Bowl

Benefits: Quinoa is a complete protein and high in fiber, making this bowl a great choice for managing diabetes and supporting digestive health.

Ingredients:

1/2 cup cooked quinoa

1/2 cup black beans, drained and rinsed

Salsa

Avocado slices

Fresh cilantro for garnish

Preparation:

Mix cooked quinoa with black beans.

Top with salsa, avocado slices, and fresh cilantro.

6. Sweet Potato and Lentil Hash

Benefits: A nutrient-dense breakfast that supports blood sugar regulation and provides essential vitamins and minerals.

Ingredients:

1 cup sweet potatoes, diced

1/2 cup cooked lentils

Red onion, diced

Spinach leaves

1 teaspoon cumin

Salt and pepper to taste

Preparation:

Sauté sweet potatoes and red onion until tender.

Add cooked lentils, spinach, cumin, salt, and pepper. Cook until spinach wilts.

7. Whole Grain Pancakes with Blueberry Compote

Benefits: These pancakes are a delicious way to incorporate whole grains and antioxidants, supporting heart health and managing cholesterol.

Ingredients:

1 cup whole wheat flour

1 tablespoon flaxseed meal

1 teaspoon baking powder

1 cup plant-based milk

Blueberry compote (simmer blueberries with a touch of maple syrup)

Preparation:

Mix whole wheat flour, flaxseed meal, baking powder, and plant-based milk until smooth.

Cook pancakes on a griddle and top with blueberry compote.

8. Green Smoothie Bowl

Benefits: Packed with greens, this smoothie bowl supports overall health, including digestion and blood pressure.

Ingredients:

1 cup spinach or kale

1/2 frozen banana

1/2 cup pineapple chunks

1/2 cup plant-based yogurt

Toppings: chia seeds, sliced banana, granola

Preparation:

Blend spinach or kale, frozen banana, pineapple, and plant-based yogurt until smooth.

Pour into a bowl and top with chia seeds, sliced banana, and granola.

9. Mediterranean Hummus Wrap

Benefits: A fiber-rich wrap that supports heart health, manages blood pressure, and provides sustained energy.

Ingredients:

Whole grain wrap

Hummus

Cucumber slices

Cherry tomatoes, halved

Kalamata olives, sliced

Fresh parsley, chopped

Preparation:

Spread hummus on a whole grain wrap.

Layer with cucumber slices, cherry tomatoes, Kalamata olives, and fresh parsley.

Roll up and enjoy.

10. Coconut and Almond Chia Pudding

Benefits: A low-fat, nutrient-dense pudding rich in omega-3 fatty acids and fiber for heart health and blood sugar control.

Ingredients:

2 tablespoons chia seeds

1/2 cup coconut milk

1/2 cup almond milk

1/2 teaspoon vanilla extract

Sliced almonds and shredded coconut for topping

Preparation:

Mix chia seeds, coconut milk, almond milk, and vanilla extract. Let it sit in the refrigerator for at least 2 hours or overnight.

Top with sliced almonds and shredded coconut before serving.

11. Cinnamon Apple Quinoa Bowl

Benefits: This breakfast bowl is a good source of fiber, antioxidants, and essential vitamins.

Ingredients:

1/2 cup cooked quinoa

1 apple, diced

1/2 teaspoon cinnamon

Plant-based yogurt for topping

Walnuts for crunch

Preparation:

Mix cooked quinoa with diced apples and cinnamon.

Top with plant-based yogurt and walnuts.

12. Tomato and Basil Avocado Toast

Benefits: A savory, low-fat option rich in antioxidants and healthy fats to support heart health.

Ingredients:

Whole grain toast

1/2 avocado, sliced

Cherry tomatoes, sliced

Fresh basil leaves

Balsamic glaze for drizzling

Preparation:

Place avocado slices on whole grain toast.

Top with sliced cherry tomatoes, fresh basil, and drizzle with balsamic glaze.

13. Vegan Banana Walnut Muffins

Benefits: These muffins offer a delicious and portable way to incorporate fiber, potassium, and omega-3 fatty acids into your breakfast.

Ingredients:

2 ripe bananas, mashed

1/4 cup maple syrup

1/4 cup plant-based milk

1 teaspoon vanilla extract

1 cup whole wheat flour

1/2 cup chopped walnuts

1 teaspoon baking powder

Preparation:

Preheat the oven to 350°F (175°C). Line a muffin tin with paper liners.

In a bowl, combine mashed bananas, maple syrup, plant-based milk, and vanilla extract.

In another bowl, whisk together whole wheat flour, chopped walnuts, and baking powder.

Add the wet ingredients to the dry ingredients and mix until just combined.

Divide the batter into the muffin cups and bake for 20-25 minutes or until a toothpick comes out clean.

14. Lentil and Vegetable Breakfast Burrito

Benefits: A protein-packed breakfast option with lentils and veggies to support blood sugar control and provide sustained energy.

Ingredients:

Whole grain tortilla

1/2 cup cooked lentils, Bell peppers, diced

Red onion, diced

Spinach leaves and Salsa for topping

Preparation:

Sauté bell peppers, red onion, and spinach until tender.

Fill a whole grain tortilla with cooked lentils and sautéed vegetables.

Top with salsa and fold into a burrito.

15. Blueberry and Almond Butter Overnight Oats

Benefits: Overnight oats are a convenient and nutritious option, providing a balance of fiber, healthy fats, and antioxidants.

Ingredients:

1/2 cup rolled oats

1/2 cup plant-based milk

1/2 cup blueberries

1 tablespoon almond butter

1 teaspoon chia seeds

Preparation:

Mix rolled oats with plant-based milk in a jar or container.

Add blueberries, almond butter, and chia seeds. Stir well.

Cover and refrigerate overnight. In the morning, give it a good stir and enjoy.

16. Mango and Coconut Chia Pudding

Benefits: A tropical delight rich in fiber, antioxidants, and healthy fats, promoting digestive health and providing sustained energy.

Ingredients:

2 tablespoons chia seeds

1/2 cup coconut milk

1/2 cup almond milk

1/2 ripe mango, diced

Shredded coconut for topping

Preparation:

Mix chia seeds, coconut milk, almond milk, and diced mango. Let it sit in the refrigerator for at least 2 hours or overnight.

Top with shredded coconut before serving.

17. Veggie and Tofu Breakfast Burrito Bowl

Benefits: A protein-packed bowl with a mix of colorful vegetables and tofu, supporting blood sugar control and providing essential nutrients.

Ingredients:

1/2 cup cooked quinoa

1/2 cup black beans, drained and rinsed

Mixed vegetables (bell peppers, zucchini, cherry tomatoes)

1/4 block firm tofu, crumbled

Salsa and cilantro for topping

Preparation:

Layer cooked quinoa with black beans, sautéed vegetables, and crumbled tofu.

Top with salsa and fresh cilantro.

18. Peanut Butter and Banana Smoothie

Benefits: A satisfying and protein-rich smoothie that supports heart health, manages blood pressure, and provides a quick energy boost.

Ingredients:

1 ripe banana

2 tablespoons peanut butter

1 cup plant-based milk

Handful of spinach

Ice cubes (optional)

Preparation:

Blend banana, peanut butter, plant-based milk, and spinach until smooth.

Add ice cubes if desired and blend again.

19. Mediterranean Quinoa Breakfast Bowl

Benefits: A savory bowl with the goodness of quinoa, olives, and vegetables, supporting heart health and providing a variety of nutrients.

Ingredients:

1/2 cup cooked quinoa

Kalamata olives, sliced

Cherry tomatoes, halved

Cucumber, diced

Hummus for topping

Preparation:

Mix cooked quinoa with sliced olives, cherry tomatoes, and diced cucumber.

Top with a dollop of hummus.

20. Pumpkin Spice Chia Seed Pudding

Benefits: A seasonal delight rich in fiber and antioxidants, promoting digestive health and providing essential nutrients.

Ingredients:

2 tablespoons chia seeds

1/2 cup pumpkin puree

1/2 teaspoon pumpkin spice

1 cup plant-based milk

Maple syrup for sweetness (optional)

Preparation:

Mix chia seeds, pumpkin puree, pumpkin spice, and plant-based milk. Let it sit in the refrigerator for at least 2 hours or overnight.

Sweeten with maple syrup if desired before serving.

CHAPTER 3: LUNCHTIME FAVORITES

1. Quinoa and Black Bean Salad

Benefits: A protein-packed salad rich in fiber and essential nutrients, supporting blood sugar control and heart health.

Ingredients:

1 cup cooked quinoa

1 cup black beans, drained and rinsed

Cherry tomatoes, halved

Cucumber, diced

Red onion, finely chopped

Fresh cilantro, chopped

Lime juice for dressing

Preparation:

Mix cooked quinoa with black beans, cherry tomatoes, cucumber, red onion, and cilantro.

Drizzle with lime juice and toss gently.

2. Lentil and Vegetable Stir-Fry

Benefits: A low-fat, high-fiber stir-fry that supports digestive health and provides plant-based protein for overall well-being.

Ingredients:

1/2 cup cooked lentils

Mixed vegetables (broccoli, bell peppers, carrots)

Garlic, minced

Low-sodium soy sauce

Brown rice for serving

Preparation:

Sauté mixed vegetables and garlic until tender.

Add cooked lentils and a splash of low-sodium soy sauce. Stir-fry until well combined.

Serve over brown rice.

3. Chickpea and Spinach Curry

Benefits: A flavorful curry rich in plant-based protein and fiber, supporting digestive health and managing blood sugar levels.

Ingredients:

1 can chickpeas, drained and rinsed

Spinach leaves

Coconut milk

Curry powder

Brown rice for serving

Preparation:

In a pot, combine chickpeas, spinach, coconut milk, and curry powder. Simmer until spinach wilts.

Serve over brown rice.

4. Sweet Potato and Black Bean Bowl

Benefits: A nutrient-dense bowl with the goodness of sweet potatoes and black beans, supporting heart health and managing blood pressure.

Ingredients:

1 cup sweet potatoes, diced

1 cup black beans, cooked

Avocado slices

Salsa

Quinoa for serving

Preparation:

Roast sweet potatoes until tender.

Mix roasted sweet potatoes with black beans.

Serve over quinoa and top with avocado slices and salsa.

5. Mediterranean Hummus Wrap

Benefits: A light and flavorful wrap providing a good source of fiber and supporting digestive health.

Ingredients:

Whole grain wrap

Hummus

Cucumber slices

Cherry tomatoes, halved

Kalamata olives, sliced

Fresh parsley, chopped

Preparation:

Spread hummus on a whole grain wrap.

Layer with cucumber slices, cherry tomatoes, Kalamata olives, and fresh parsley.

Roll up and enjoy.

6. Brown Rice and Vegetable Sushi Rolls

Benefits: Low in fat and rich in fiber, these sushi rolls provide a delicious way to incorporate vegetables and whole grains into your diet.

Ingredients:

Nori sheets

Brown rice, cooked

Carrots, julienned

Cucumber, julienned

Avocado slices

Soy sauce for dipping

Preparation:

Place a nori sheet on a bamboo sushi mat.

Spread a thin layer of cooked brown rice over the nori.

Add julienned carrots, cucumber, and avocado slices.

Roll tightly and slice into sushi rolls. Serve with soy sauce.

7. Broccoli and Chickpea Buddha Bowl

Benefits: A nutrient-dense bowl with broccoli and chickpeas, providing fiber and supporting digestive health.

Ingredients:

Steamed broccoli florets

1 cup cooked chickpeas

Quinoa

Lemon-tahini dressing

Preparation:

Arrange steamed broccoli and cooked chickpeas over quinoa.

Drizzle with lemon-tahini dressing.

8. Spinach and Lentil Salad with Balsamic Vinaigrette

Benefits: A refreshing salad rich in iron, fiber, and antioxidants, supporting heart health and digestion.

Ingredients:

2 cups baby spinach

1/2 cup cooked lentils

Cherry tomatoes, halved

Red onion, thinly sliced

Balsamic vinaigrette dressing

Preparation:

Toss baby spinach with cooked lentils, cherry tomatoes, and thinly sliced red onion.

Drizzle with balsamic vinaigrette dressing.

9. Cauliflower and Chickpea Curry

Benefits: A flavorful and low-fat curry with cauliflower and chickpeas, supporting digestive health and providing plant-based protein.

Ingredients:

1/2 head cauliflower, chopped

1 can chickpeas, drained and rinsed, Coconut milk

Curry powder and Brown rice for serving.

Preparation:

In a pot, combine cauliflower, chickpeas, coconut milk, and curry powder. Simmer until cauliflower is tender.

Serve over brown rice.

10. Mexican Quinoa Bowl

Benefits: A protein-rich bowl with quinoa and black beans, supporting blood sugar control and providing essential nutrients.

Ingredients:

1 cup cooked quinoa

1 cup black beans, cooked

Corn kernels

Avocado slices

Salsa

Fresh cilantro, chopped

Preparation:

Mix cooked quinoa with black beans, corn kernels, and fresh cilantro.

Top with avocado slices and salsa.

11. Eggplant and Chickpea Stew

Benefits: A hearty stew rich in fiber and plant-based protein, supporting digestive health and overall well-being.

Ingredients:

1 eggplant, diced

1 can chickpeas, drained and rinsed

Tomato sauce

Garlic, minced

Fresh basil, chopped

Whole grain couscous for serving

Preparation:

Sauté diced eggplant and minced garlic until eggplant is tender.

Add chickpeas, tomato sauce, and fresh basil. Simmer until flavors meld.

Serve over whole grain couscous.

12. Avocado and Black Bean Wrap

Benefits: A satisfying and fiber-rich wrap with the goodness of avocados and black beans, supporting heart health and digestion.

Ingredients:

Whole grain wrap

1/2 avocado, mashed

1 cup black beans, cooked

Salsa

Spinach leaves

Preparation:

Spread mashed avocado on a whole grain wrap.

Layer with black beans, salsa, and spinach leaves.

Roll up and enjoy.

13. Roasted Vegetable Quinoa Bowl

Benefits: A colorful and nutrient-dense bowl with roasted vegetables and quinoa, supporting digestive health and providing essential vitamins.

Ingredients:

Assorted vegetables (bell peppers, zucchini, cherry tomatoes)

1 cup cooked quinoa

Balsamic glaze

Fresh herbs for garnish

Preparation:

Roast assorted vegetables until tender.

Arrange roasted vegetables over cooked quinoa.

Drizzle with balsamic glaze and garnish with fresh herbs.

14. Spaghetti Squash Primavera

Benefits: A low-calorie alternative to traditional pasta, rich in fiber and antioxidants, supporting weight management and digestive health.

Ingredients:

Roasted spaghetti squash

Mixed vegetables (bell peppers, cherry tomatoes, broccoli)

Marinara sauce

Fresh basil, chopped

Preparation:

Scrape roasted spaghetti squash into strands.

Sauté mixed vegetables until tender and toss with spaghetti squash.

Top with marinara sauce and chopped fresh basil.

15. Asparagus and Red Lentil Soup

Benefits: A warming soup rich in fiber and plant-based protein, supporting digestive health and providing essential nutrients.

Ingredients:

1 bunch asparagus, chopped

1 cup red lentils, rinsed

Vegetable broth

Garlic, minced

Lemon juice for garnish

Preparation:

In a pot, combine chopped asparagus, red lentils, vegetable broth, and minced garlic. Simmer until lentils are tender.

Garnish with a squeeze of lemon juice before serving.

16. Mediterranean Quinoa Salad

Benefits: A refreshing salad loaded with quinoa and colorful vegetables, providing fiber and supporting heart health.

Ingredients:

1 cup cooked quinoa

Cherry tomatoes, halved

Cucumber, diced

Kalamata olives, sliced

Red onion, finely chopped

Fresh parsley, chopped

Olive oil and lemon juice for dressing

Preparation:

Mix cooked quinoa with cherry tomatoes, cucumber, Kalamata olives, red onion, and fresh parsley.

Drizzle with olive oil and lemon juice. Toss gently before serving.

17. Teriyaki Tofu Stir-Fry

Benefits: A protein-packed stir-fry with tofu and colorful vegetables, supporting blood sugar control and providing essential nutrients.

Ingredients:

Firm tofu, cubed

Mixed vegetables (broccoli, bell peppers, snap peas)

Low-sodium teriyaki sauce

Brown rice for serving

Preparation:

Sauté cubed tofu until golden brown.

Add mixed vegetables and teriyaki sauce. Stir-fry until vegetables are tender.

Serve over brown rice.

18. Cauliflower and Lentil Tacos

Benefits: A flavorful and low-fat taco filling with cauliflower and lentils, providing plant-based protein and supporting digestive health.

Ingredients:

1/2 head cauliflower, finely chopped

1 cup cooked green or brown lentils

Taco seasoning

Whole grain tortillas

Salsa and guacamole for topping

Preparation:

Sauté cauliflower and cooked lentils with taco seasoning until well combined.

Serve the mixture in whole grain tortillas and top with salsa and guacamole.

19. Chickpea and Vegetable Buddha Bowl

Benefits: A nutrient-dense bowl with chickpeas and colorful vegetables, supporting digestive health and providing essential vitamins and minerals.

Ingredients:

1 cup cooked chickpeas

Roasted sweet potatoes

Steamed broccoli florets

Shredded carrots

Quinoa

Tahini dressing

Preparation:

Arrange cooked chickpeas, roasted sweet potatoes, steamed broccoli, and shredded carrots over quinoa.

Drizzle with tahini dressing.

20. Zucchini Noodles with Pesto

Benefits: A low-calorie, high-fiber alternative to traditional pasta, rich in nutrients and supporting weight management.

Ingredients:

Zucchini, spiralized into noodles

Cherry tomatoes, halved

Pine nuts

Fresh basil pesto (homemade or store-bought)

Preparation:

Sauté zucchini noodles until just tender.

Toss with cherry tomatoes and pine nuts.

Drizzle with fresh basil pesto before serving.

CHAPTER 4: SATISFYING DINNER

1. Lentil and Vegetable Stuffed Bell Peppers

Benefits: Fiber-rich lentils combined with colorful vegetables make this dish a low-fat option supporting digestive health and managing blood sugar levels.

Ingredients:

Bell peppers, halved

1 cup cooked green or brown lentils

Mixed vegetables (zucchini, carrots, tomatoes)

Tomato sauce

Herbs and spices for seasoning

Preparation:

Sauté mixed vegetables until tender.

Mix vegetables with cooked lentils and seasonings.

Stuff bell peppers with the lentil-vegetable mixture and bake until peppers are soft.

2. Chickpea and Spinach Curry

Benefits: A flavorful curry with chickpeas and spinach, rich in fiber and plant-based protein, supporting digestive health and blood sugar control.

Ingredients:

1 can chickpeas, drained and rinsed

Spinach leaves

Coconut milk

Curry powder

Brown rice for serving

Preparation:

In a pot, combine chickpeas, spinach, coconut milk, and curry powder. Simmer until spinach wilts.

Serve over brown rice.

3. Quinoa and Black Bean Casserole

Benefits: Protein-packed quinoa and black beans combined with vegetables create a satisfying, low-fat casserole supporting heart health and digestion.

Ingredients:

1 cup cooked quinoa

1 can black beans, drained and rinsed

Corn kernels

Diced bell peppers

Tomato sauce

Cumin and chili powder for seasoning

Preparation:

Mix cooked quinoa with black beans, corn, bell peppers, and seasoning.

Layer the mixture in a casserole dish and bake until heated through.

4. Sweet Potato and Chickpea Curry

Benefits: A nutrient-dense curry with sweet potatoes and chickpeas, providing fiber and supporting blood sugar regulation.

Ingredients:

Sweet potatoes, diced

1 can chickpeas, drained and rinsed

Coconut milk

Curry spices (turmeric, cumin, coriander)

Brown rice for serving

Preparation:

Sauté sweet potatoes until slightly tender.

Add chickpeas, coconut milk, and curry spices. Simmer until sweet potatoes are fully cooked.

Serve over brown rice.

5. Vegetable and Lentil Stir-Fry

Benefits: A quick and flavorful stir-fry with a mix of vegetables and lentils, providing plant-based protein and supporting digestive health.

Ingredients:

Mixed vegetables (broccoli, bell peppers, snap peas)

1 cup cooked green or brown lentils

Low-sodium soy sauce

Brown rice for serving

Preparation:

Sauté mixed vegetables until crisp-tender.

Add cooked lentils and a splash of low-sodium soy sauce. Stir-fry until well combined.

Serve over brown rice.

6. Mediterranean Quinoa Bowl

Benefits: A light and refreshing bowl with quinoa and Mediterranean flavors, supporting heart health and providing essential nutrients.

Ingredients:

1 cup cooked quinoa

Cherry tomatoes, halved

Cucumber, diced

Kalamata olives, sliced

Red onion, finely chopped

Fresh parsley, chopped

Olive oil and lemon juice for dressing

Preparation:

Mix cooked quinoa with cherry tomatoes, cucumber, Kalamata olives, red onion, and fresh parsley.

Drizzle with olive oil and lemon juice. Toss gently before serving.

7. Zucchini Noodles with Tomato Sauce

Benefits: A low-calorie alternative to traditional pasta, zucchini noodles are paired with a homemade tomato sauce, providing fiber and supporting weight management.

Ingredients:

Zucchini, spiralized into noodles

Tomato sauce (homemade or low-fat store-bought)

Fresh basil, chopped

Garlic, minced

Preparation:

Sauté zucchini noodles until just tender.

Heat tomato sauce with minced garlic.

Toss zucchini noodles with tomato sauce and top with fresh basil.

8. Cauliflower and Chickpea Salad

Benefits: A crunchy and satisfying salad with roasted cauliflower and chickpeas, providing fiber and supporting digestive health.

Ingredients:

1/2 head cauliflower, chopped

1 can chickpeas, drained and rinsed

Mixed greens

Cherry tomatoes, halved

Lemon-tahini dressing

Preparation:

Roast cauliflower and chickpeas until golden brown.

Arrange roasted cauliflower and chickpeas over mixed greens.

Drizzle with lemon-tahini dressing.

9. Eggplant and Quinoa Bake

Benefits: A hearty bake featuring eggplant and quinoa, providing fiber and supporting digestive health.

Ingredients:

Eggplant, sliced

1 cup cooked quinoa

Tomato sauce

Basil and oregano for seasoning

Nutritional yeast (optional)

Preparation:

Layer sliced eggplant in a baking dish.

Mix cooked quinoa with tomato sauce, basil, and oregano. Spread over the eggplant.

Bake until the eggplant is tender. Sprinkle with nutritional yeast if desired.

10. Butternut Squash and Lentil Stew

Benefits: A comforting stew with butternut squash and lentils, providing fiber and supporting blood sugar regulation.

Ingredients:

Butternut squash, diced

1 cup green or brown lentils

Vegetable broth

Onion, chopped

Garlic, minced

Sage and thyme for seasoning

Preparation:

Sauté onion and garlic until softened.

Add diced butternut squash, lentils, vegetable broth, sage, and thyme. Simmer until lentils are tender.

11. Spinach and Mushroom Quinoa Risotto

Benefits: A nutrient-dense twist on traditional risotto with quinoa, spinach, and mushrooms, providing fiber and essential nutrients.

Ingredients:

1 cup cooked quinoa

Spinach leaves

Mushrooms, sliced

Vegetable broth

Nutritional yeast (optional)

Lemon zest for garnish

Preparation:

Sauté mushrooms until tender.

Add cooked quinoa, spinach, and vegetable broth. Simmer until spinach wilts.

Sprinkle with nutritional yeast and garnish with lemon zest.

12. Chickpea and Vegetable Skewers

Benefits: Grilled chickpea and vegetable skewers are a flavorful and low-fat option, providing plant-based protein and supporting digestive health.

Ingredients:

1 can chickpeas, drained and rinsed

Mixed vegetables (bell peppers, zucchini, cherry tomatoes)

Olive oil and herbs for marinating

Preparation:

Marinate chickpeas and vegetables in olive oil and herbs.

Thread onto skewers and grill until vegetables are tender.

13. Tomato and Basil Zoodles

Benefits: Light and refreshing, this dish features zucchini noodles with a tomato and basil sauce, providing fiber and supporting weight management.

Ingredients:

Zucchini, spiralized into noodles

Cherry tomatoes, halved

Fresh basil, chopped

Garlic, minced

Olive oil for sautéing

Preparation:

Sauté zucchini noodles in olive oil until just tender.

Add cherry tomatoes, minced garlic, and fresh basil. Cook until tomatoes are softened.

14. Black Bean and Corn Stuffed Portobello Mushrooms

Benefits: Stuffed portobello mushrooms with black beans and corn provide a satisfying, low-fat option rich in fiber and essential nutrients.

Ingredients:

Portobello mushrooms, cleaned

1 can black beans, drained and rinsed

Corn kernels and Salsa for topping

Preparation:

Remove stems from portobello mushrooms.

Mix black beans and corn. Stuff into the mushrooms.

Bake until mushrooms are tender. Top with salsa before serving.

15. Mediterranean Chickpea and Artichoke Salad

Benefits: A refreshing salad with chickpeas and artichokes, providing fiber and supporting heart health.

Ingredients:

1 can chickpeas, drained and rinsed

Artichoke hearts, chopped

Cherry tomatoes, halved

Cucumber, diced

Kalamata olives, sliced

Feta cheese (optional)

Olive oil and lemon juice for dressing

Preparation:

Mix chickpeas with artichoke hearts, cherry tomatoes, cucumber, and Kalamata olives.

If using, crumble feta cheese over the salad.

Drizzle with olive oil and lemon juice. Toss gently before serving.

16. Spaghetti Squash Primavera

Benefits: A low-calorie alternative to traditional pasta, this dish features spaghetti squash with a medley of colorful vegetables, providing fiber and supporting weight management.

Ingredients:

Roasted spaghetti squash

Mixed vegetables (bell peppers, cherry tomatoes, broccoli)

Marinara sauce

Fresh basil, chopped

Preparation:

Scrape roasted spaghetti squash into strands.

Sauté mixed vegetables until tender and toss with spaghetti squash.

Top with marinara sauce and chopped fresh basil.

17. Broccoli and Tofu Stir-Fry

Benefits: A quick and flavorful stir-fry with broccoli and tofu, providing plant-based protein and supporting digestive health.

Ingredients:

Broccoli florets

Firm tofu, cubed

Low-sodium soy sauce

Ginger and garlic, minced

Brown rice for serving

Preparation:

Sauté cubed tofu until golden brown.

Add broccoli, ginger, garlic, and a splash of low-sodium soy sauce. Stir-fry until broccoli is tender.

Serve over brown rice.

18. Stuffed Acorn Squash with Quinoa and Cranberries

Benefits: A festive dish with acorn squash stuffed with quinoa and cranberries, providing fiber and supporting heart health.

Ingredients:

Acorn squash, halved

1 cup cooked quinoa

Dried cranberries

Pecans, chopped

Maple syrup for drizzling

Preparation:

Roast acorn squash halves until tender.

Mix cooked quinoa with dried cranberries and chopped pecans.

Stuff the acorn squash with the quinoa mixture and drizzle with maple syrup.

19. Cauliflower and Lentil Tacos

Benefits: Flavorful and low-fat taco filling with cauliflower and lentils, providing plant-based protein and supporting digestive health.

Ingredients:

1/2 head cauliflower, finely chopped

1 cup cooked green or brown lentils

Taco seasoning

Whole grain tortillas

Salsa and guacamole for topping

Preparation:

Sauté cauliflower and cooked lentils with taco seasoning until well combined.

Serve the mixture in whole grain tortillas and top with salsa and guacamole.

20. Greek Salad with Quinoa and Chickpeas

Benefits: A refreshing Greek salad with the added protein of quinoa and chickpeas, providing fiber and supporting heart health.

Ingredients:

1 cup cooked quinoa

Chickpeas, drained and rinsed

Cherry tomatoes, halved

Cucumber, diced

Red onion, finely chopped

Kalamata olives, sliced

Feta cheese (optional)

Greek dressing

Preparation:

Mix cooked quinoa with chickpeas, cherry tomatoes, cucumber, red onion, and Kalamata olives.

If using, crumble feta cheese over the salad.

Drizzle with Greek dressing. Toss gently before serving.

CHAPTER 5: SNACKS AND APPETIZER

1. Edamame Hummus with Veggie Sticks

Benefits: A protein-packed hummus made with edamame, paired with fresh vegetable sticks for a satisfying and fiber-rich snack.

Ingredients:

1 cup cooked edamame

1 clove garlic, minced

Lemon juice

Olive oil

Carrot and cucumber sticks for dipping

Preparation:

Blend edamame, garlic, lemon juice, and olive oil until smooth.

Serve with carrot and cucumber sticks.

2. Roasted Chickpeas

Benefits: Crunchy and high in fiber, roasted chickpeas make a flavorful and low-fat snack, perfect for managing cholesterol.

Ingredients:

1 can chickpeas, drained and rinsed

Olive oil

Smoked paprika

Cumin

Garlic powder

Preparation:

Toss chickpeas with olive oil and seasonings.

Roast in the oven until crispy.

3. Guacamole with Whole Grain Pita Chips

Benefits: Avocados in guacamole provide healthy fats, while whole grain pita chips add fiber for a heart-healthy snack.

Ingredients:

Ripe avocados

Tomatoes, diced

Red onion, finely chopped

Lime juice

Whole grain pita, cut into wedges

Preparation:

Mash avocados and mix with tomatoes, red onion, and lime juice.

Bake whole grain pita wedges until crispy. Serve with guacamole.

4. Berry and Chia Seed Pudding

Benefits: Chia seeds are rich in fiber, and combined with berries, this pudding is a delicious, low-fat option to support heart health.

Ingredients:

2 tablespoons chia seeds

Plant-based milk

Mixed berries

Maple syrup (optional)

Preparation:

Mix chia seeds with plant-based milk and let it sit until it thickens.

Layer with mixed berries. Sweeten with maple syrup if desired.

5. Veggie Spring Rolls with Peanut Dipping Sauce

Benefits: Packed with fresh vegetables, these spring rolls are a light and fiber-rich snack, and the peanut sauce adds healthy fats.

Ingredients:

Rice paper wrappers

Cabbage, shredded

Carrots, julienned

Cucumber, thinly sliced

Fresh mint leaves

Peanut butter for the dipping sauce

Preparation:

Dip rice paper wrappers in warm water to soften.

Fill with cabbage, carrots, cucumber, and mint. Roll tightly.

Mix peanut butter with a bit of water for the dipping sauce.

6. Sliced Apple with Almond Butter

Benefits: Apples provide fiber, while almond butter adds healthy fats and protein for a satisfying and heart-healthy snack.

Ingredients:

Apples, sliced

Almond butter

Preparation:

Spread almond butter on apple slices.

7. Mediterranean Chickpea Salad

Benefits: A refreshing salad with chickpeas, tomatoes, and cucumbers, offering fiber and supporting digestive health.

Ingredients:

1 can chickpeas, drained and rinsed

Cherry tomatoes, halved

Cucumber, diced

Red onion, finely chopped

Kalamata olives, sliced

Olive oil and lemon juice

Preparation:

Mix chickpeas with tomatoes, cucumber, red onion, and Kalamata olives.

Drizzle with olive oil and lemon juice.

8. Stuffed Mini Bell Peppers

Benefits: Colorful mini bell peppers stuffed with a flavorful mix of beans and vegetables make for a tasty and fiber-filled snack.

Ingredients:

Mini bell peppers, halved

Black beans, mashed

Corn kernels

Salsa

Preparation:

Fill mini bell pepper halves with mashed black beans and corn.

Top with salsa.

9. Kale Chips

Benefits: A crunchy and low-fat alternative to potato chips, kale chips are rich in fiber and antioxidants.

Ingredients:

Kale leaves, torn into pieces

Olive oil

Nutritional yeast (optional)

Preparation:

Toss kale with olive oil and nutritional yeast.

Bake until crisp.

10. Cucumber and Hummus Bites

Benefits: Cucumber slices paired with hummus create a refreshing and satisfying snack, rich in fiber and supporting digestive health.

Ingredients:

Cucumber, sliced

Hummus

Preparation:

Spread hummus on cucumber slices.

11. Avocado Salsa

Benefits: Avocados provide healthy fats, and combined with tomatoes and onions, this salsa is a tasty and fiber-rich option.

Ingredients:

Ripe avocados, diced

Tomatoes, diced

Red onion, finely chopped

Cilantro, chopped

Lime juice

Preparation:

Mix diced avocados with tomatoes, red onion, cilantro, and lime juice.

12. Quinoa Stuffed Mushrooms

Benefits: Quinoa is a good source of fiber, and when stuffed into mushrooms, it makes for a nutritious and low-fat appetizer.

Ingredients:

Mushrooms, cleaned and stemmed

Cooked quinoa

Spinach, chopped

Garlic, minced

Preparation:

Sauté garlic and spinach. Mix with cooked quinoa.

Stuff mushrooms with the quinoa mixture. Bake until mushrooms are tender.

13. Baked Sweet Potato Fries

Benefits: Sweet potatoes offer fiber and essential nutrients, and when baked, they make for a delicious and low-fat snack.

Ingredients:

Sweet potatoes, cut into fries

Olive oil

Paprika

Cumin

Preparation:

Toss sweet potato fries with olive oil, paprika, and cumin.

Bake until crispy.

14. Spinach and Artichoke Dip with Whole Grain Crackers

Benefits: This classic dip made with spinach and artichokes is paired with whole grain crackers for a tasty and fiber-rich appetizer.

Ingredients:

Frozen spinach, thawed and drained

Artichoke hearts, chopped

Vegan cream cheese

Whole grain crackers

Preparation:

Mix thawed spinach with chopped artichoke hearts and vegan cream cheese.

Serve with whole grain crackers.

15. Baked Falafel with Tahini Sauce

Benefits: Chickpea-based falafel is baked for a low-fat option, and served with tahini sauce for a flavorful and fiber-rich snack.

Ingredients:

Canned chickpeas, drained

Onion, chopped

Fresh herbs (parsley, cilantro)

Whole wheat pita for serving

Tahini sauce

Preparation:

Blend chickpeas, chopped onion, and fresh herbs until a dough form.

Form into balls and bake until golden brown.

Serve with whole wheat pita and tahini sauce.

CHAPTER 6: SWEET DESSERT

1. Mixed Berry Chia Seed Pudding

Benefits: Chia seeds provide fiber, while mixed berries offer natural sweetness, making this pudding a delicious and heart-healthy dessert.

Ingredients:

2 tablespoons chia seeds

Plant-based milk

Mixed berries

Maple syrup (optional)

Preparation:

Mix chia seeds with plant-based milk and let it sit until it thickens.

Layer with mixed berries. Sweeten with maple syrup if desired.

2. Baked Apples with Cinnamon

Benefits: Apples are rich in fiber, and when baked with cinnamon, they create a satisfying and low-fat dessert.

Ingredients:

Apples, cored and sliced

Cinnamon

Nutmeg

Oats (optional)

Preparation:

Arrange apple slices in a baking dish.

Sprinkle with cinnamon and nutmeg. Bake until tender.

Top with oats if desired.

3. Banana-Oat Cookies

Benefits: These cookies use bananas and oats, providing fiber and a naturally sweet flavor without added sugar.

Ingredients:

Ripe bananas, mashed

Rolled oats

Cinnamon

Nuts or seeds (optional)

Preparation:

Mix mashed bananas with rolled oats and cinnamon.

Fold in nuts or seeds if desired.

Drop spoonful onto a baking sheet and bake until golden.

4. Avocado Chocolate Mousse

Benefits: Avocados contribute healthy fats, and when blended with cocoa, they create a rich and creamy chocolate mousse.

Ingredients:

Ripe avocados

Cocoa powder

Maple syrup or agave nectar

Preparation:

Blend avocados, cocoa powder, and sweetener until smooth.

Chill before serving.

5. Quinoa Pudding with Almond Milk

Benefits: Quinoa adds protein and fiber to this creamy pudding made with almond milk, creating a nutritious and low-fat dessert.

Ingredients:

Cooked quinoa

Almond milk

Vanilla extract

Cinnamon

Raisins (optional)

Preparation:

Mix cooked quinoa with almond milk, vanilla extract, and cinnamon.

Stir in raisins if desired. Chill before serving.

6. Peach and Berry Sorbet

Benefits: This refreshing sorbet is made with peaches and berries, providing vitamins and antioxidants in a low-fat and naturally sweet treat.

Ingredients:

Peaches, sliced

Mixed berries

Lemon juice

Maple syrup (optional)

Preparation:

Blend peaches and berries with lemon juice.

Sweeten with maple syrup if desired.

Freeze until firm.

7. Pumpkin Spice Energy Bites

Benefits: Pumpkin adds fiber to these energy bites, creating a satisfying and flavorful treat without added sugars.

Ingredients:

Canned pumpkin puree

Rolled oats

Pumpkin spice

Almond butter

Chia seeds

Preparation:

Mix pumpkin puree, oats, pumpkin spice, almond butter, and chia seeds.

Form into bite-sized balls and chill.

8. Berry Parfait with Coconut Yogurt

Benefits: Coconut yogurt adds creaminess to this parfait, while berries provide fiber and antioxidants for a delightful and healthy dessert.

Ingredients:

Coconut yogurt

Mixed berries

Granola (low-fat)

Preparation:

Layer coconut yogurt with mixed berries and low-fat granola.

9. Mango and Coconut Chia Popsicles

Benefits: These popsicles combine the tropical flavors of mango and coconut with chia seeds for added fiber and a refreshing, low-fat treat.

Ingredients:

Mango, diced

Coconut milk

Chia seeds

Preparation:

Blend mango with coconut milk.

Stir in chia seeds and pour into popsicle molds. Freeze until solid.

10. Chocolate-Dipped Strawberries

Benefits: Strawberries are high in fiber and antioxidants, and when dipped in dark chocolate, they make for a decadent and heart-healthy dessert.

Ingredients:

Strawberries

Dark chocolate (70% cocoa or higher)

Preparation:

Melt dark chocolate.

Dip each strawberry into the melted chocolate. Allow to set.

11. Blueberry Oat Bars

Benefits: These bars are made with oats and blueberries, providing fiber and antioxidants in a satisfying and low-fat dessert.

Ingredients:

Rolled oats

Blueberries

Applesauce

Cinnamon

Preparation:

Mix rolled oats with blueberries, applesauce, and cinnamon.

Press into a baking dish and bake until set.

12. Watermelon and Mint Salad

Benefits: Watermelon is hydrating and low in calories, while mint adds a refreshing twist to create a light and healthy dessert.

Ingredients:

Watermelon, cubed

Fresh mint leaves

Lime juice

Preparation:

Toss watermelon cubes with fresh mint leaves.

Drizzle with lime juice before serving.

13. Cinnamon-Roasted Butternut Squash

Benefits: Butternut squash is rich in fiber and vitamins, and when roasted with cinnamon, it becomes a sweet and low-fat dessert.

Ingredients:

Butternut squash, peeled and cubed

Cinnamon

Nutmeg

Maple syrup (optional)

Preparation:

Toss butternut squash with cinnamon and nutmeg.

Roast until tender. Sweeten with maple syrup if desired.

14. Vegan Chocolate Avocado Pudding

Benefits: Avocado adds creaminess to this vegan chocolate pudding, creating a satisfying and low-fat dessert rich in antioxidants.

Ingredients:

Ripe avocados

Cocoa powder

Coconut milk

Maple syrup

Preparation:

Blend avocados, cocoa powder, coconut milk, and maple syrup until smooth.

Chill before serving.

15. Apricot and Almond Bliss Balls

Benefits: Dried apricots and almonds provide fiber and natural sweetness in these bliss balls, offering a satisfying and nutritious dessert.

Ingredients:

Dried apricots

Almonds

Shredded coconut

Vanilla extract

Preparation:

Blend dried apricots, almonds, shredded coconut, and vanilla extract until a dough form.

Roll into small balls and chill.

16. Pomegranate and Pistachio Yogurt Parfait

Benefits: Pomegranate seeds and pistachios add crunch and flavor to this yogurt parfait, offering a nutrient-rich and low-fat dessert.

Ingredients:

Plant-based yogurt

Pomegranate seeds

Pistachios, chopped

Drizzle of honey (optional)

Preparation:

Layer plant-based yogurt with pomegranate seeds and chopped pistachios.

Drizzle with honey if desired.

17. Date and Walnut Energy Balls

Benefits: Dates and walnuts create a naturally sweet and nutty energy ball, providing fiber and a satisfying treat.

Ingredients:

Dates, pitted

Walnuts

Chia seeds

Coconut flakes

Preparation:

Blend dates and walnuts until a sticky mixture form.

Form into small balls and roll in chia seeds and coconut flakes.

18. Raspberry and Almond Chia Seed Pudding

Benefits: Raspberries and almonds add vibrant flavors to this chia seed pudding, creating a delicious and fiber-rich dessert.

Ingredients:

Chia seeds

Almond milk

Raspberries

Sliced almonds

Preparation:

Mix chia seeds with almond milk and let it sit until thickened.

Layer with fresh raspberries and sliced almonds.

19. Coconut and Pineapple Sorbet

Benefits: This tropical sorbet is made with coconut and pineapple, offering a refreshing and low-fat dessert with natural sweetness.

Ingredients:

Coconut milk

Pineapple, diced

Lime juice

Agave syrup (optional)

Preparation:

Blend coconut milk with diced pineapple and lime juice.

Sweeten with agave syrup if desired.

Freeze until firm.

20. Almond Butter Stuffed Dates

Benefits: Stuffed dates with almond butter provide a sweet and satisfying dessert rich in fiber and healthy fats.

Ingredients:

Medjool dates, pitted

Almond butter

Sea salt (optional)

Preparation:

Fill each date with a spoonful of almond butter.

Sprinkle with sea salt if desired.

CHAPTER 7: SPECIAL OCCASION MENUS

1. Quinoa-Stuffed Bell Peppers

Benefits: Quinoa provides protein and fiber, and when stuffed into bell peppers, it creates a colorful and nutritious dish suitable for special occasions.

Ingredients:

Bell peppers, halved

Cooked quinoa

Black beans

Corn

Salsa for topping

Preparation:

Mix cooked quinoa with black beans and corn.

Stuff bell peppers and bake until tender.

Top with salsa before serving.

2. Lentil and Vegetable Curry

Benefits: Lentils offer plant-based protein and fiber, while the rich vegetable curry adds flavor, making this dish perfect for special occasions.

Ingredients:

Lentils, cooked

Mixed vegetables (carrots, peas, spinach)

Coconut milk

Curry spices

Preparation:

Sauté mixed vegetables and cooked lentils in curry spices.

Stir in coconut milk and simmer until vegetables are tender.

3. Eggplant and Chickpea Tagine

Benefits: Eggplant and chickpeas create a hearty and fiber-rich tagine, making it a flavorful option for special occasions.

Ingredients:

Eggplant, diced

Chickpeas, cooked

Tomatoes

Moroccan spices

Preparation:

Sauté diced eggplant and cooked chickpeas in Moroccan spices.

Add tomatoes and simmer until flavors meld.

4. Spinach and Mushroom Stuffed Portobello Mushrooms

Benefits: Spinach and mushrooms provide vitamins and fiber in this elegant stuffed portobello mushroom dish for special occasions.

Ingredients:

Portobello mushrooms, cleaned

Spinach, chopped

Mushrooms, diced

Garlic, minced

Preparation:

Sauté chopped spinach, diced mushrooms, and minced garlic.

Stuff portobello mushrooms and bake until tender.

5. Cauliflower and Chickpea Shawarma Wraps

Benefits: Cauliflower and chickpeas make a delicious and fiber-filled shawarma filling for wraps, perfect for special occasions.

Ingredients:

Cauliflower, roasted

Chickpeas, roasted

Whole grain wraps

Tahini sauce

Preparation:

Roast cauliflower and chickpeas with shawarma spices.

Fill whole grain wraps with the roasted mixture and drizzle with tahini sauce.

6. Butternut Squash and Sage Risotto

Benefits: Butternut squash adds sweetness and fiber to this creamy sage-infused risotto, creating an elegant dish for special occasions.

Ingredients:

Arborio rice

Butternut squash, diced

Vegetable broth

Fresh sage leaves

Preparation:

Sauté Arborio rice and diced butternut squash in olive oil.

Gradually add vegetable broth and stir until creamy.

Garnish with fresh sage leaves.

7. Vegan Lentil Loaf

Benefits: A hearty lentil loaf made with vegetables and spices, offering a plant-based, high-fiber alternative for special occasions.

Ingredients:

Lentils, cooked

Carrots, grated

Oats

Tomato sauce

Vegan Worcestershire sauce

Preparation:

Mix cooked lentils, grated carrots, oats, tomato sauce, and Worcestershire sauce.

Shape into a loaf and bake until firm.

8. Sweet Potato and Black Bean Enchiladas

Benefits: Sweet potatoes and black beans create a flavorful and fiber-rich enchilada filling, perfect for special occasions.

Ingredients:

Sweet potatoes, mashed

Black beans, cooked

Whole grain tortillas

Enchilada sauce

Preparation:

Mix mashed sweet potatoes with cooked black beans.

Fill whole grain tortillas, roll, and top with enchilada sauce.

9. Artichoke and Spinach Stuffed Mushrooms

Benefits: Artichokes and spinach combine to create a tasty and fiber-filled stuffing for mushrooms, ideal for special occasions.

Ingredients:

Mushrooms, cleaned

Artichoke hearts, chopped

Spinach, chopped

Vegan cream cheese

Preparation:

Sauté chopped artichoke hearts and spinach. Mix with vegan cream cheese.

Stuff mushrooms and bake until tender.

10. Mediterranean Quinoa Salad

Benefits: Quinoa, olives, and vegetables make a refreshing and fiber-rich Mediterranean salad, perfect for special occasions.

Ingredients:

Quinoa, cooked

Cherry tomatoes, halved

Cucumber, diced

Kalamata olives, sliced

Red onion, finely chopped

Olive oil and lemon juice

Preparation:

Mix cooked quinoa with cherry tomatoes, cucumber, Kalamata olives, and red onion.

Drizzle with olive oil and lemon juice. Toss gently before serving.

11. Zucchini Noodles with Pesto

Benefits: Zucchini noodles tossed with basil pesto create a light and flavorful dish, perfect for special occasions.

Ingredients:

Zucchini noodles

Basil pesto

Cherry tomatoes, halved

Pine nuts

Preparation:

Sauté zucchini noodles and toss with basil pesto.

Top with cherry tomatoes and pine nuts before serving.

12. Roasted Brussels Sprouts and Quinoa Bowl

Benefits: Roasted Brussels sprouts and quinoa create a hearty bowl packed with fiber and nutrients, suitable for special occasions.

Ingredients:

Brussels sprouts, halved

Quinoa, cooked

Balsamic glaze

Toasted almonds

Preparation:

Roast halved Brussels sprouts until caramelized.

Serve over cooked quinoa and drizzle with balsamic glaze. Top with toasted almonds.

13. Stuffed Acorn Squash with Wild Rice and Cranberries

Benefits: Acorn squash stuffed with wild rice and cranberries offers a festive and fiber-rich dish for special occasions.

Ingredients:

Acorn squash, halved

Wild rice, cooked

Dried cranberries

Pecans, chopped

Maple syrup for drizzling

Preparation:

Roast acorn squash halves until tender.

Mix cooked wild rice with dried cranberries and chopped pecans.

Stuff the acorn squash and drizzle with maple syrup.

14. Vegan Mushroom Wellington

Benefits: A plant-based mushroom Wellington with flaky pastry and a savory filling, making it an impressive centerpiece for special occasions.

Ingredients:

Portobello mushrooms

Puff pastry

Spinach, chopped

Vegan cream cheese

Preparation:

Sauté chopped spinach and mix with vegan cream cheese.

Place portobello mushrooms on puff pastry, add the spinach mixture, and encase in the pastry.

Bake until golden brown.

15. Coconut and Berry Chia Seed Parfait

Benefits: Chia seeds provide fiber, and when layered with coconut yogurt and berries, they create a visually appealing and nutritious parfait for special occasions.

Ingredients:

Chia seeds

Coconut yogurt

Mixed berries

Granola (low-fat)

Preparation:

Mix chia seeds with coconut yogurt and let it sit until thickened.

Layer with mixed berries and low-fat granola.

CONCLUSION

This High Fiber Vegetarian Diet Cookbook serves as an invaluable guide for individuals seeking to embrace a health-conscious lifestyle through a high-fiber diet. The carefully curated recipes within these pages not only cater to the nutritional needs of those managing conditions such as diabetes, high cholesterol, high blood pressure, and IBS but also offer a delectable journey into the world of plant-based, low-fat culinary delights.

This cookbook is not merely a compilation of recipes, it is a special companion on the journey to enhanced well-being. Through a thoughtfully crafted table of contents, the cookbook effortlessly guides readers through a diverse array of breakfasts, lunches, dinners, snacks, appetizers, desserts, and special occasion dishes. Each section not only provides flavorful recipes but also offers insight into the benefits of incorporating high-fiber, plant-based foods into one's diet.

The introduction sets the tone by illustrating the adverse effects of a low-fiber diet on the body, creating an immediate awareness of the importance of embracing a more fiber-rich lifestyle. It emphasizes the transformative power of a plant-based diet, not only for physical health but also for overall well-being.

For those grappling with specific health concerns, such as diabetes, high cholesterol, high blood pressure, or IBS, this cookbook stands out as a tailored resource. The meticulously crafted recipes take into account dietary restrictions and preferences, ensuring that individuals can indulge in delicious meals without compromising their health goals.

The breakfast, lunch, and dinner recipes showcase the versatility and abundance of plant-based ingredients. From the vibrant Mediterranean Quinoa Salad to the comforting Butternut Squash and Sage Risotto, each dish is a testament to the notion that healthy eating can be a flavorful and satisfying experience.

The inclusion of snacks and appetizers like the Guacamole with Whole Grain Pita Chips and the Berry and Chia Seed Pudding adds an element of enjoyment to daily eating habits. These snacks not only curb cravings but also contribute to the overall goal of maintaining a balanced, high-fiber diet.

Desserts take center stage with creative options like the Avocado Chocolate Mousse and the Blueberry Oat Bars. These sweet treats prove that indulgence can be guilt-free and that desserts can be both delicious and health-promoting.

Finally, for special occasions, the cookbook offers a collection of recipes that elevate plant-based dining to a sophisticated level. From the elegant Stuffed Acorn Squash with Wild Rice and Cranberries to the show-stopping Vegan Mushroom Wellington, these dishes emphasize that high-fiber eating can be a celebration of taste and health.

In essence, this High Fiber Vegetarian Diet Cookbook goes beyond being a mere collection of recipes, it is a guide, a companion, and a source of inspiration for those embarking on a journey toward a high-fiber, plant-based lifestyle. It is a celebration of the vibrant and diverse world of vegetarian cuisine, proving that nourishing the body and delighting the palate can go hand in hand. With its wealth of information, enticing recipes, and a focus on holistic well-being, this cookbook is a special guide for anyone aspiring to embrace the benefits of a high-fiber diet.

Happy Cooking!

4-WEEK MEAL PLANNER

WEEK 1:

WEEKLY MEAL PLANNER

START DATE _____   END DATE _____

MONDAY

TUESDAY

WEDNESDAY

THURSDAY

FRIDAY

SATURDAY

SUNDAY

SHOPPING LIST
- _____
- _____
- _____
- _____
- _____
- _____
- _____

COMMENT

WEEK 2:

WEEKLY MEAL PLANNER

START DATE _____   END DATE _____

MONDAY

TUESDAY

WEDNESDAY

THURSDAY

FRIDAY

SATURDAY

SUNDAY

SHOPPING LIST
- ○ _____
- ○ _____
- ○ _____
- ○ _____
- ○ _____
- ○ _____
- ○ _____

COMMENT

WEEK 3:

WEEKLY (MEAL PLANNER)

START DATE _____   END DATE _____

MONDAY

SATURDAY

TUESDAY

SUNDAY

WEDNESDAY

SHOPPING LIST
- ○ _____
- ○ _____
- ○ _____
- ○ _____
- ○ _____
- ○ _____
- ○ _____

THURSDAY

COMMENT

FRIDAY

WEEK 4:

WEEKLY MEAL PLANNER

START DATE _____ END DATE _____

MONDAY

TUESDAY

WEDNESDAY

THURSDAY

FRIDAY

SATURDAY

SUNDAY

SHOPPING LIST
- ○ _____
- ○ _____
- ○ _____
- ○ _____
- ○ _____
- ○ _____
- ○ _____

COMMENT

Printed in Great Britain
by Amazon

43715740R00069